GLUTEN FREE

FOOD LIST

The World's Most Comprehensive Ingredient List for
the Gluten-Free Diet - Take It Wherever You Go!

LEGAL & DISCLAIMER

resulting from the application of any of the information provided by this guide. This disclaimer applies to any damages or injury caused by the use and application, whether directly or indirectly, of any advice or information presented, whether for breach of contract, tort, negligence, personal injury, criminal intent, or under any other cause of action. You agree to accept all risks of using the information presented inside this book.

CONTENTS

LEGAL & DISCLAIMER 1

CONTENTS 3

INTRODUCTION.. 19

HOW TO USE THIS FOOD LIST 21

LEGAL DEFINITIONS OF 'GLUTEN-FREE'.. 23

SOURCES... 25

DISCLAIMER 27

THE FOOD LIST 29

    acerola 29

    agave syrup 29

    alcohol... 29

    alcoholic beverages... 29

    algae and algae derivatives 29

    almond... 30

    all non-organic meat is suspect, especially if aged 30

    amaranth... 30

    anchovies.. 30

    anise, aniseed 30

    apple 30

    apple cider vinegar.. 30

apricot...31
artichoke...31
artificial sweeteners 31
Asimina triloba...31
asparagus 31
aubergine 31
avocado 31
bamboo shoots...31
banana...32
Barbary fig 32
barley 32
barley malt, malt...32
basil 32
bay laurel, laurel 32
beans (pulses)...32
beef (depending on age of beef, organic, freshly cooked).....32
beef (fresh) 33
beer 33
beetroot..33
bell pepper (hot) 33
bell pepper (sweet)...33
bison (organic, freshly cooked)..33
bivalves (mussels, oyster, clams, scallops)........................33
black caraway..33
black caraway oil 34
blackberry...34
blackcurrants 34
blue cheeses, mold cheeses..34

blue fenugreek..34
blueberries..34
bok choi...34
borlotti beans..34
bouillon (yeast extract / meat extract / glutamate)..............35
boysenberry..35
brandy...35
Brazil nut..35
bread...35
broad bean..35
broad-leaved garlic..35
broccoli...35
brown algae, algae...36
brussels sprouts...36
buckrams...36
buckwheat...36
Butter..36
Butterkaese...36
buttermilk..36
cabbage, green or white...37
cactus pear..37
caraway...37
cardamom...37
carrot...37
cashew nut..37
cassava..37
cassava flour...37
cauliflower...38

celery..38
celery cabbage 38
cep 38
chamomile tea 38
champagne..38
chard stalks 38
chayote 38
cheddar cheese..39
cheese made from unpasteurised "raw" milk.......................39
cheese: soft cheeses 39
cheese: hard cheese, all well matured cheeses....................39
cherry..39
chestnut, sweet chestnut 39
chia 40
Chicken 40
chickpeas 40
chicory..40
chili pepper, red, fresh..40
chives 40
chocolate 40
cilantro...41
cinnamon...41
citrus fruits 41
clover..41
cloves 41
cocoa butter 41
cocoa drinks 41
cocoa, cocoa powder (chocolate, etc.) 42

coconut fat, coconut oil 42
coconut, coconut shavings, coconut milk........................ 42
Coffee... 42
Cola-drinks 42
common sea-buckthorn 42
coriander 42
corn 43
corn salad, lamb's lettuce.. 43
cornflakes (if no additives) 43
courgette 43
cowberry... 43
crab 44
cranberry 44
cranberry nectar.. 44
crawfish 44
cream cheeses (means: very young cheeses), plain,
without additives 44
cream, sweet, without additives 44
cress: garden cress.. 44
cucumber 45
cumin 45
curd cheese 45
curry 45
dates (dried, desiccated).. 45
dextrose.. 45
dill... 45
distilled white vinegar 46
dog rose.. 46

dragon fruit, pitaya..46
dried meat (any kind)...46
dry-cured ham 46
duck...46
earth almond 46
egg white 47
egg yolk...47
eggplant...47
eggs, chicken egg, whole egg 47
elderflower cordial 47
elderflower cordial 47
endive 47
energy drinks 47
entrails..48
espresso (see blog on coffee) 48
ethanol..48
ewe's milk, sheep's milk...48
extract of malt..48
farmer's cheese (a type of fresh cheese)......................48
fennel 48
fennel flower (Nigella sativa).......................................49
fennel flower oil (Nigella sativa)...................................49
fenugreek 49
Feta cheese 49
figs (fresh or dried)...49
fish (freshly caught within an hour or frozen within
an hour) 49
fish (in the shop in the cooling rack or on ice)...............49

Flaxseed (linseed) 50
Fontina cheese 50
Fries, chips 50
fructose (fruit sugar) 50
game 50
garden cress 50
garlic (usually well tolerated) 51
Geheimratskaese, Geheimrats cheese 51
German turnip 51
ginger 51
glucose 51
goat's milk, goat milk 51
goji berry, Chinese wolfberry, Chinese boxthorn,
Himalayan goji, Tibetan goji 51
goose (organic, freshly cooked) 51
gooseberry, gooseberries 52
Gouda cheese (young) 52
Gouda cheese, old 52
gourds 52
grapefruit 52
grapes 52
gravy 52
green algae, algae 53
green beans 53
green peas 53
green split peas 53
green tea 53
guava 53

ham (dried, cured)..53

hazelnut..54

hemp seeds (Cannabis sativa) 54

herbal teas with medicinal herbs 54

honey 54

horseradish...54

hot chocolate 54

Indian fig opuntia, Barbary fig, cactus pear, spineless
cactus, prickly pear, tuna..54

innards...54

inverted sugar syrup 55

ispaghula, psyllium seed husks 55

Jeera (Cumin)...55

Jostaberry 55

Juniper Berries 55

Kaki (Persimmon) 55

Kale..55

Kefir 56

Kelp (Large Seaweeds, Algae)...56

Kelp, Seaweed, Algae 56

Khorasan Wheat 56

Kiwi Fruit...56

Kohlrabi 56

Kombu Seaweed..56

Lactose (Milk Sugar) 57

Ladyfinger Banana 57

Lamb (Organic, Freshly Cooked)..57

Lamb's Lettuce, Corn Salad 57

Langouste 57
Lard 57
Laurel, Bay Laurel, Sweet Bay, Bay Tree, True Laurel,
Grecian Laurel 57
Leek 58
Lemon 58
Lemon Peel, Lemon Zest 58
Lemonade 58
Lentils 58
Lettuce Iceberg 58
Lettuce: Head and Leaf Lettuces 58
Lime 58
Lime Blossom Tea, Limeflower, Flowers of Large-Leaved
Limetree 59
Lingonberry 59
Liquor, Clear 59
Liquor, Schnapps, Spirits, Cloudy (Not Colourless) 59
Liquorice Root 59
Lobster 59
Loganberry 59
Lychee 60
Macadamia 60
Malt Extract 60
Malt, Barley Malt 60
Maltodextrin 60
Maltose, Malt Sugar (Pure) 60
Mandarin Orange 60
Mango 61

Maple Syrup 61
Margarine 61
Marrow 61
Mascarpone Cheese... 61
Mate Tea 61
Meat Extract 61
Melons (Except Watermelon)... 62
Meridian Fennel.. 62
Milk, Lactose-free 62
Milk, Pasteurised 62
Milk, UHT 62
Milk powder 62
Millet 62
Minced Meat (If Eaten Immediately After Its Production) 62
Minced Meat (Open Sale or Pre-Packed)............................ 63
Mineral water, still... 63
Mint 63
Mold cheeses, mould cheeses 63
Morel 63
Morello cherries.. 63
Mozzarella cheese 63
Mulberry 64
Mungbeans (germinated, sprouting) 64
Mushrooms, different types 64
Mustard, mustard seeds, mustardseed powder 64
Napa cabbage 64
Nashi pear 64
Nectarine 64

Nigella sativa oil 64
Nigella sativa seed 65
Nori seaweed 65
Nut grass 65
Nutmeg 65
Nutmeg flower 65
Nutmeg flower oil 65
Nuts 65
Oat drink, oat milk 66
Oats 66
Olive oil 66
Olives 66
Onion 66
Orange 66
Orange juice 67
Orange peel, orange zest 67
Oregano 67
Ostrich 67
Ostrich (organic, freshly cooked) 67
Oyster 67
Pak choi 67
Palm kernel oil 67
Palm oil, dendê oil 67
Palm sugar 68
Papaya, pawpaw 68
Paprika, hot 68
Paprika, sweet 68
Parsley 68

Parsnip 68
Passionfruit 68
Pasta (search individual ingredients, eg wheat, corn) 68
Paw paw 69
Peach 69
Peanuts 69
Pear 69
Pear, peeled canned in sugar syrup 69
Pearl sago 69
Peas (green) 70
Pea shoots 70
Pepper, black 70
Pepper, white 70
Peppermint tea 70
Perennial wall-rocket 70
Persian cumin 70
Persimmon 70
Pickled cabbage 71
Pickled cucumber 71
Pickled gherkin 71
Pickled vegetables 71
Pine nuts 71
Pineapple 71
Pistachio 71
Pitaya, pitahaya, dragon fruit 72
Pizza base (search individual ingredients,
eg wheat, corn) 72
Plaice 72

Plantains 72
Plum 72
Pomegranate 72
Pomegranate juice 72
Popcorn (plain, popped) 73
Poppyseed.. 73
Porcini mushrooms.. 73
Pork 73
Pork (organic, freshly cooked) 73
Portabello mushrooms.. 73
Potato... 73
Potato flour 73
Potato starch... 74
Prunes 74
Pumpkin.. 74
Pumpkin seeds 74
Quail... 74
Quince.. 74
Quinoa 74
Quinoa flakes 74
Rabbit... 75
Radicchio 75
Radish 75
Raisins 75
Rapeseed oil.. 75
Raspberries 75
Red cabbage.. 75
Red onions... 75

Red pepper, bell pepper 75
Redcurrants 76
Reindeer 76
Rice 76
Rice bran oil 76
Rice cakes 76
Rice flour 76
Rice milk 76
Rice noodles 77
Rice paper 77
Rice vinegar 77
Rosemary 77
Runner beans 77
Rutabaga, swede 77
Rye 77
Safflower oil 78
Saffron 78
Sage 78
Salmon 78
Sardines 78
Sauerkraut 78
Scallop 78
Sea bass 78
Sea bream 79
Seafood (fresh, unprocessed) 79
Seaweed 79
Sesame oil 79
Sesame seeds 79

Shallots 79
Sheep 79
Shiitake mushrooms 79
Shrimp 80
Skimmed milk 80
Sloe berries 80
Smoked fish (plain, no additives)................................... 80
Smoked meat (plain, no additives) 80
Soba noodles 80
Sorbet... 80
Sorghum 81
Sorghum flour 81
Soy sauce 81
Spaghetti squash 81
Spinach 81
Split peas 81
Squash (all varieties) 82
Star anise.. 82
Stevia.. 82
Strawberries.. 82
Sugar (white, brown, confectioner's)............................. 82
Sunflower oil 82
Sunflower seeds 82
Sweet potatoes 82
Swiss chard... 83
Tangerines... 83
Tapioca.. 83
Tapioca flour 83

Tarragon 83

Tea 83

Thyme 83

Tofu 84

Tomatillos 84

Tomatoes 84

Trout 84

Tuna (fresh) 84

Turkey (fresh, unprocessed) 84

Turmeric 84

Turnips 85

Vanilla extract 85

Venison 85

Vinegar (distilled white, balsamic, wine, apple cider) 85

Walnuts 85

Watercress 85

Wheat 85

Wheatgrass 86

Whitefish 86

Wild rice 86

Wine 86

Xanthan gum 86

Yams 87

Yogurt (plain, unflavored) 87

Zucchini 87

CASE STUDIES 89

INTRODUCTION

We are so pleased to help you on your gluten-free journey. This book has been a passion project to put together. It's something we needed and wanted ourselves. We, too, have had our battles with food intolerances and sensitivities, with gluten being our particular problem. Over the course of decades of being gluten-free, we've made every mistake it's possible to make. That's why we've put particular emphasis on potential stumbling blocks in this book; suspect sauces, gluten-containing gravies, fries that are listed as gluten-free on a menu but cooked in the same oil as a million other gluten-containing items - we've got your back.

And let us tell you, the sea of information out there can often seem as clear as mud. Who'd have thought that gluten, the stuff that makes breads and pastas so delightfully chewy, could cause so much trouble?

And trouble, it does. This is precisely why we have taken the initiative to compile our own comprehensive list of gluten-free foods, drawing from the most reliable and trusted gluten guides available. The conflicting opinions and contradictory information surrounding gluten content in various food items can be likened to observing a tennis match, where experts present divergent viewpoints, leaving us perplexed as to whether a bagel, for instance, should be considered a friend or a foe in terms of gluten content. To address this uncertainty, we have chosen to confront the issue head-on and create a meticulously crafted catalog of foods, ensuring accuracy and consistency.

In plain English, gluten is a group of proteins found in wheat, barley, and rye. Think of it as the glue that helps food keep its shape. The catch? For some of us, this protein can wreak havoc in our bodies, causing everything from a mildly upset tummy to severe autoimmune reactions.

We all react to gluten in different ways, which is why there's so much debate about what foods are safe and what aren't. That's where this book comes in. It's like your gluten-free compass, helping you navigate through the fog.

Things like wheat, rye, and barley are the usual suspects, and easy to spot. Other things may be harder, so take this book everywhere. Ready to dive in? Let's get this gluten-free show on the road!

HOW TO USE THIS FOOD LIST

Think of this book as your gluten-free dictionary. It's got an alphabetized list of foods, drinks, and ingredients you can flip through or search with ease.

We've sifted through the world's best resources and boiled down all that information into a simple rating system. Each item gets a score from 0 to 2, based on its gluten content.

Here's the breakdown:

0 - Generally safe. These foods are gluten-free. (Though still check labels, be aware of cross contamination and potential errors)

1 - Extreme caution. There is debate around these foods, or they sometimes contain gluten. Proceed with caution.

2 - Red alert! These are high in gluten and best avoided.

In the grand scheme of things, a score of 0 is great, and a score of 2 is a big red flag and very likely to contain gluten. Over time, with guidance from your healthcare provider, you can figure out which foods hit the right notes and which ones fall flat.

Remember, this is a guide. The real key to nailing your gluten-free diet is understanding your body. So let this book be your sidekick as you embark on your gluten-free adventure. Whether you're whipping up a meal at home or dining out, let it help you make smarter, healthier choices. Keep it handy, and you're good to go!

LEGAL DEFINITIONS OF 'GLUTEN-FREE'.

By law, in the U.S. and in many other countries, a food product can only be labeled "gluten-free" if it contains less than 20 parts per million (ppm) of gluten.

Now, you're probably thinking, "Wait a minute, that means there's still gluten in there!" And you'd be absolutely right. Let's put this into context with an example. Picture this: if you took one million grains of rice, and only 20 of those grains were gluten, that's the equivalent of 20ppm. It's a teeny tiny amount, but it's not zero.

So, even when a product says "gluten-free" on the label, it could technically contain minute traces of gluten. If you're particularly sensitive to gluten or have been diagnosed with celiac disease, this could potentially be an issue. We've come across plenty of people for whom this is an issue.

For example: Some beers are labeled "gluten-removed" or "gluten-reduced." These are made with traditional gluten-containing grains, but an enzyme is added during the brewing process that breaks down the gluten. These beers might meet the legal definition of "gluten-free" in that they contain less than 20ppm of gluten, but there's still debate in the medical community about whether these are safe for people with celiac disease or severe gluten intolerance. We say: avoid.

Hard liquor, such as vodka, gin, or whiskey, is another area where confusion can arise. These spirits are often distilled from grains like wheat, barley, or rye. But here's the thing - the distillation process should technically remove all gluten proteins, making the final product safe for people on a gluten-free diet.

However, just as with our food example earlier, there can be traces of gluten present due to potential cross-contamination in the manufacturing process. So, a vodka or a whiskey could potentially contain up to 20ppm of gluten, even if it's labeled as "gluten-free."

We say: it's confusing. Some of our writers can tolerate certain alcohols distilled from grains, others cannot tolerate any. Whisky is a particular culprit. If there's any doubt whatsoever, avoid.

Remember that everyone's sensitivity to gluten is different, and what works for one person might not work for another. If you have any doubts, it's best to consult with your healthcare provider.

SOURCES

These excellent sources come highly recommended in your further research on gluten.

Please check out these top gluten information sites for further reading. We consider them to be the best sources out there.

1. [Celiac Disease Foundation](https://celiac.org): This organization offers a wealth of information about celiac disease and gluten-free living. They provide comprehensive lists of foods and ingredients to avoid and those that are safe to eat.

2. [Gluten-Free Living](https://www.glutenfreeliving.com): This website and magazine provide practical advice, recipes, and tips for living gluten-free.

3. [National Celiac Association](https://nationalceliac.org): The NCA offers numerous resources for understanding and managing celiac disease and gluten sensitivities, including a comprehensive list of gluten-free foods.

4. [Gluten Intolerance Group](https://gluten.org): A leading source of consumer and industry information on gluten-free standards and labeling.

5. [Beyond Celiac](https://www.beyondceliac.org): This organization provides a multitude of resources for people with celiac disease and gluten sensitivity, including lists of gluten-free foods and potential sources of hidden gluten.

6. [The Gluten-Free Society](https://www.glutenfreesociety.org): The Gluten-Free Society is a comprehensive resource for all things gluten-free. They provide food lists, as well as research and education on gluten sensitivity and celiac disease.

7. [Coeliac UK](https://www.coeliac.org.uk): An excellent resource for those living in the UK, Coeliac UK provides extensive lists of gluten-free foods, recipes, and tips for living a gluten-free lifestyle.

8. [Verywell Fit](https://www.verywellfit.com): Verywell Fit provides resources on various diets, including gluten-free. They offer lists of foods to avoid and those that are safe to eat.

9. [Mayo Clinic](https://www.mayoclinic.org): Mayo Clinic has an extensive collection of resources on celiac disease and gluten-free diets, including food lists, recipes, and tips for managing a gluten-free lifestyle.

10. [American Dietetic Association](https://www.eatright.org): Their resources offer a comprehensive understanding of the gluten-free diet, from knowing what to avoid, how to read labels, to planning gluten-free meals.

DISCLAIMER

The creation of this book has entailed an immense amount of dedication, perseverance, and, on occasion, even emotional investment. However, it is important to acknowledge that we are not medical professionals donning lab coats, nor do we possess an authoritative monopoly on what constitutes optimal nourishment for your body. This is where the expertise of your healthcare provider becomes indispensable.

We emphatically stress the necessity of consulting with your doctor, dietitian, or healthcare provider before implementing any modifications to your dietary regimen. These individuals possess the invaluable expertise and personalized insights required to offer you tailored advice and guidance. Their professional knowledge and support make them the true champions in safeguarding your well-being.

Next, let's talk about food labels. These little guys are your secret weapon in your gluten-free journey. Manufacturers often change their recipes, and a food that was gluten-free yesterday might not be gluten-free today. So, make sure to check food labels every single time, even if it's a product you've bought a million times before. We've made those gluten mistakes too many times.

Finally, while we've made every effort to make sure our gluten scores are as accurate as possible, remember that they're not set in stone. Different people react to gluten in different ways. Sometimes something is labelled as gluten-free because it meets a legal definition of gluten-free (for example, the ppm definition we already looked at), but it doesn't suit you and you react to it. What's fine for one person might cause problems for another. So, always listen to your body and take things at your own pace.

In short, think of this book as your gluten-free BFF. It's here to lend a hand, offer advice, and help you make sense of it all. But at the end of the day, it's just a guide, not a replacement for professional medical advice or your own good judgment.

To reiterate: The information contained in this book has been compiled from sources deemed reliable, and it is accurate to the best of the Author's knowledge; however, the Author cannot guarantee its accuracy and validity and cannot be held liable for any errors or omissions.

Now, let's get this gluten-free adventure started!

The Food List

acerola - 0

Acerola is a fruit and naturally gluten-free.

agave syrup - 0

Agave syrup is derived from a plant and is naturally gluten-free.

alcohol - 2

Some alcohols are gluten-free (see individual alcohols) but owing to the distillation process there is often significant amounts of gluten in alcohol and so this is too broad to score anything else but 2.

alcoholic beverages - 2

Like alcohol, many alcoholic beverages can contain gluten, especially those made from wheat, barley, and rye. Always check labels.

algae and algae derivatives - 0

Algae and its derivatives are plant-based and naturally gluten-free.

almond - 0

Almonds are naturally gluten-free, but be cautious of cross-contamination in processed products.

all non-organic meat is suspect, especially if aged - 1

While meat is naturally gluten-free, processing, flavorings, or cross-contamination can introduce gluten. Cooked chicken in stores - for example - often has gluten injected into it to bulk it up (doesn't sound very appetising does it.)

amaranth - 0

Amaranth is a naturally gluten-free grain.

anchovies - 0

Anchovies are a type of fish and are naturally gluten-free. However, some preparations or brands may contain gluten.

anise, aniseed - 0

Anise is a plant and naturally gluten-free.

apple - 0

Apples are naturally gluten-free.

apple cider vinegar - 0

Apple cider vinegar is made from apples, and it's gluten-free.

apricot - 0

Apricots are naturally gluten-free.

artichoke - 0

Artichokes are naturally gluten-free.

artificial sweeteners - 1

While many artificial sweeteners are gluten-free, some may contain gluten due to the additives used. Always check the label.

Asimina triloba - 0

Also known as pawpaw, Asimina triloba is a fruit and is naturally gluten-free.

asparagus - 0

Asparagus is naturally gluten-free.

aubergine - 0

Also known as eggplant, aubergines are naturally gluten-free.

avocado - 0

Avocados are naturally gluten-free.

bamboo shoots - 0

Bamboo shoots are naturally gluten-free.

banana - 0

Bananas are naturally gluten-free.

Barbary fig - 0

Also known as prickly pear, Barbary figs are naturally gluten-free.

barley - 2

Barley is a gluten-containing grain and should be avoided.

barley malt, malt - 2

Barley malt and malt are derived from barley, a gluten-containing grain. These should be avoided.

basil - 0

Basil is naturally gluten-free.

bay laurel, laurel - 0

Bay laurel is a plant and is naturally gluten-free.

beans (pulses) - 0

Beans are naturally gluten-free. However, cross-contamination can occur in processing facilities, so always check labels.

beef (depending on age of beef, organic, freshly cooked) - 1

While beef is naturally gluten-free, processed or flavored beef products may contain gluten. Always check labels.

beef (fresh) - 0

Fresh beef is naturally gluten-free.

beer - 2

Most beer is made from malted barley and contains gluten, although gluten-free beers are now available.

beetroot - 0

This root vegetable is naturally gluten-free.

bell pepper (hot) - 0

These peppers are naturally gluten-free.

bell pepper (sweet) - 0

Sweet bell peppers are naturally gluten-free.

bison (organic, freshly cooked) - 0

This meat is naturally gluten-free, provided it is fresh and cooked without gluten-containing additives.

bivalves (mussels, oyster, clams, scallops) - 0

These seafoods are naturally gluten-free, but be aware of sauces and preparation methods that may introduce gluten.

black caraway - 0

This spice is naturally gluten-free.

black caraway oil - 0

The oil derived from black caraway is naturally gluten-free.

blackberry - 0

This fruit is naturally gluten-free.

blackcurrants - 0

Blackcurrants are naturally gluten-free.

blue cheeses, mold cheeses - 1

These cheeses can contain gluten due to cross-contamination in the aging process.

blue fenugreek - 0

This spice is naturally gluten-free.

blueberries - 0

Blueberries are naturally gluten-free.

bok choi - 0

This vegetable is naturally gluten-free.

borlotti beans - 0

These beans are naturally gluten-free, but check for cross-contamination in processing.

bouillon (yeast extract / meat extract / glutamate) - 2

Many bouillon cubes and powders contain gluten in the form of wheat flour or wheat starch, or through additives.

boysenberry - 0

Boysenberries are naturally gluten-free.

brandy - 2

Brandy is a distilled alcohol that can potentially contain gluten due to distillation from gluten grains.

Brazil nut - 0

Brazil nuts are naturally gluten-free, but check for cross-contamination in processing.

bread - 2

Most bread is made from wheat flour and thus contains gluten, but gluten-free breads are available.

broad bean - 0

Broad beans are naturally gluten-free.

broad-leaved garlic - 0

This herb is naturally gluten-free.

broccoli - 0

Broccoli is naturally gluten-free.

brown algae, algae - 0

This food is naturally gluten-free, but it's always a good idea to check the labels for added gluten in any form.

brussels sprouts - 0

Brussels sprouts are naturally gluten-free.

buckrams - 0

This plant is naturally gluten-free.

buckwheat - 0

Despite its name, buckwheat is not a type of wheat and is naturally gluten-free, but check for cross-contamination in processing.

Butter - 1

Butter is naturally gluten-free, but flavored or spreadable versions may contain gluten.

Butterkaese - 0

Butterkaese is a type of cheese and is generally gluten-free, but check labels to be sure.

buttermilk - 0

Buttermilk is naturally gluten-free, but check labels to ensure no gluten-containing additives are included.

cabbage, green or white - 0

Cabbage is naturally gluten-free.

cactus pear - 0

Cactus pear, also known as prickly pear, is naturally gluten-free.

caraway - 0

Caraway seeds are naturally gluten-free.

cardamom - 0

This spice is naturally gluten-free.

carrot - 0

Carrots are naturally gluten-free.

cashew nut - 0

Cashews are naturally gluten-free, but check for cross-contamination in processing.

cassava - 0

Cassava is a root vegetable that is naturally gluten-free. It's a great gluten-free flour alternative which we love to cook with.

cassava flour - 0

Cassava flour is made from the gluten-free cassava root. See above - one of our favourite gluten free flours.

cauliflower - 0

Cauliflower is naturally gluten-free.

celery - 0

Celery is naturally gluten-free.

celery cabbage - 0

This vegetable is naturally gluten-free.

cep - 0

Cep is a type of mushroom that is naturally gluten-free.

chamomile tea - 0

Pure chamomile tea is naturally gluten-free, but check labels as some flavored or blended teas may contain gluten.

champagne - 2

Champagne is a type of wine, and while the grapes are gluten-free, the fining process can introduce trace amounts of gluten. Which is something we didn't know. Check with your supplier.

chard stalks - 0

Chard is a type of vegetable that is naturally gluten-free.

chayote - 0

Chayote is a type of squash that is naturally gluten-free.

cheddar cheese - 0

Cheddar cheese is typically gluten-free, but some brands may introduce gluten during processing, so always check the label.

cheese made from unpasteurised "raw" milk - 0

Cheese made from raw milk is typically gluten-free, but it is always a good idea to check the labels for any added ingredients that may contain gluten.

cheese: soft cheeses - 0

Soft cheeses are typically gluten-free. As with any cheese, it is always best to check the label for any gluten-containing additives.

cheese: hard cheese, all well matured cheeses - 0

Hard, well-matured cheeses are typically gluten-free, but again, always check the label for any gluten-containing additives.

cherry - 0

Cherries are naturally gluten-free.

chestnut, sweet chestnut - 0

Chestnuts are naturally gluten-free.

chia - 0

Chia seeds are naturally gluten-free.

Chicken - 0

Chicken is naturally gluten-free, provided it is cooked without any gluten-containing additives. As noted above, cooked chicken often contains gluten either in a glaze or in the chicken itself. As long as the chicken has not been prepared or cooked with gluten-containing ingredients, it is gluten-free.

chickpeas - 0

Chickpeas are naturally gluten-free.

chicory - 0

Chicory is naturally gluten-free.

chili pepper, red, fresh - 0

Fresh red chili peppers are naturally gluten-free.

chives - 0

Chives are naturally gluten-free.

chocolate - 1

Some chocolate, especially milk and white chocolate, can contain gluten due to additives or cross-contamination during production. Some cheaper chocolate brands 'fill out' their chocolate with gluten-containing ingredients. Check individual brands.

cilantro - 0

Cilantro, also known as coriander in some regions, is naturally gluten-free.

cinnamon - 0

Cinnamon is naturally gluten-free.

citrus fruits - 0

Citrus fruits, including oranges, lemons, limes, and grapefruits, are naturally gluten-free.

clover - 0

Clover is naturally gluten-free.

cloves - 0

Cloves are naturally gluten-free.

cocoa butter - 0

Cocoa butter is naturally gluten-free.

cocoa drinks - 1

Cocoa drinks can sometimes contain gluten due to additives or cross-contamination in production, so always check the label.

cocoa, cocoa powder (chocolate, etc.) - 0

Pure cocoa and cocoa powder are naturally gluten-free, but always check labels as some brands may add gluten-containing additives.

coconut fat, coconut oil - 0

Coconut fat and coconut oil are naturally gluten-free.

coconut, coconut shavings, coconut milk - 0

Coconuts, coconut shavings, and coconut milk are all naturally gluten-free.

Coffee - 0

Plain coffee is naturally gluten-free, but flavored coffees and additives may contain gluten.

Cola-drinks - 1

Cola drinks may contain caramel color or barley malt, which can occasionally contain gluten. It's always best to check the label.

common sea-buckthorn - 0

Sea-buckthorn is naturally gluten-free.

coriander - 0

Coriander is naturally gluten-free.

corn - 0

Corn is naturally gluten-free, but beware of cross-contamination, especially when eating out or eating processed foods. Beware of products like 'cornflakes' - it would be reasonable to think cornflakes are only made of corn, but that's not necessarily the case - see below.

corn salad, lamb's lettuce - 0

Corn salad, also known as lamb's lettuce, is naturally gluten-free.

cornflakes (if no additives) - 1

Plain cornflakes would be typically gluten-free, but many brands add malt flavoring or other additives that contain gluten. Always check the label. For example, Kellogg's Corn Flakes have gluten in them. Even though the main ingredient is milled corn, the cereal also contains barley malt extract, which has gluten in it.

courgette - 0

Courgette, also known as zucchini, is naturally gluten-free.

cowberry - 0

Cowberries, also known as lingonberries, are naturally gluten-free.

crab - 0

Crab is naturally gluten-free, but beware of sauces and preparation methods that may introduce gluten.

cranberry - 0

Cranberries are naturally gluten-free.

cranberry nectar - 0

Cranberry nectar is typically gluten-free, but always check the label for any gluten-containing additives.

crawfish - 0

Crawfish, also known as crayfish, are naturally gluten-free, but beware of sauces and preparation methods that may introduce gluten.

cream cheeses (means: very young cheeses), plain, without additives - 0

Cream cheeses are generally gluten-free, but flavored or spreadable versions may contain gluten.

cream, sweet, without additives - 0

Sweet cream without additives is gluten-free.

cress: garden cress - 0

Garden cress is naturally gluten-free.

cucumber - 0

Cucumbers are naturally gluten-free.

cumin - 0

Cumin is naturally gluten-free.

curd cheese - 0

Curd cheese is typically gluten-free, but check labels to be sure.

curry - 1

Curry is a blend of spices, all of which should be gluten-free. However, often there will be some sort of gluten-containing ingredient in there, so check carefully. Also be aware of potential cross-contamination during processing.

dates (dried, desiccated) - 0

Dates are naturally gluten-free, but check labels to ensure no gluten-containing additives or cross-contamination.

dextrose - 0

Dextrose, a type of sugar, is naturally gluten-free.

dill - 0

Dill is naturally gluten-free.

distilled white vinegar - 0

Distilled white vinegar is typically gluten-free. Vinegar made from gluten grains can be a source of gluten, but the distillation process should remove any gluten.

dog rose - 0

Dog rose, a type of wild rose, is naturally gluten-free.

dragon fruit, pitaya - 0

Dragon fruit, also known as pitaya, is naturally gluten-free.

dried meat (any kind) - 1

Dried meats can sometimes contain gluten due to additives or flavorings, so always check the label.

dry-cured ham - 0

Dry-cured ham is typically gluten-free, but check labels to ensure no gluten-containing additives are used.

duck - 0

Duck is naturally gluten-free, provided it is prepared and cooked without gluten-containing ingredients.

earth almond - 0

Earth almonds, also known as tiger nuts, are naturally gluten-free.

egg white - 0

Egg whites are naturally gluten-free.

egg yolk - 0

Egg yolks are naturally gluten-free.

eggplant - 0

Eggplant, also known as aubergine, is naturally gluten-free.

eggs, chicken egg, whole egg - 0

Eggs are naturally gluten-free.

elderflower cordial - 1

Elderflower cordial can

elderflower cordial - 1

Elderflower cordial can sometimes contain gluten due to additives or processing methods. Always check the label to be sure.

endive - 0

Endive is naturally gluten-free.

energy drinks - 1

Many energy drinks can contain gluten due to added ingredients or cross-contamination during manufacturing. Always check labels.

entrails - 0

Entrails, or offal, from animals are naturally gluten-free, but be aware of how they are prepared and cooked.

espresso (see blog on coffee) - 0

Espresso is naturally gluten-free, but flavored espressos and additives may contain gluten.

ethanol - 0

Ethanol itself is gluten-free, but be cautious as it can be derived from gluten-containing grains.

ewe's milk, sheep's milk - 0

Sheep's milk is naturally gluten-free.

extract of malt - 2

Malt extract is typically made from barley, a gluten-containing grain, so it is not safe for those with celiac disease or gluten intolerance.

farmer's cheese (a type of fresh cheese) - 0

Farmer's cheese is typically gluten-free, but check labels to be sure.

fennel - 0

Fennel is naturally gluten-free.

fennel flower (Nigella sativa) - 0

Fennel flower is naturally gluten-free.

fennel flower oil (Nigella sativa) - 0

Fennel flower oil is naturally gluten-free.

fenugreek - 0

Fenugreek is naturally gluten-free.

Feta cheese - 0

Feta cheese is typically gluten-free, but check labels to be sure.

figs (fresh or dried) - 0

Figs are naturally gluten-free.

fish (freshly caught within an hour or frozen within an hour) - 0

Fish is naturally gluten-free, provided it is not prepared with gluten-containing ingredients.

fish (in the shop in the cooling rack or on ice) - 0

Fish from a store should also be gluten-free, but always check for any added ingredients, especially in pre-seasoned or marinated varieties.

Flaxseed (linseed) - 0

Flaxseed is naturally gluten-free, but as with all seeds, it's best to look for versions labeled gluten-free to avoid cross-contamination.

Fontina cheese - 0

Fontina cheese is typically gluten-free, but check labels to be sure.

Fries, chips - 1

In theory, if potato fries are made from one ingredient (potatoes) then they are gluten-free. But in practice fries are often a) coated with a gluten-containing ingredient or b) cooked in oil which has already cooked lots of other gluten-containing foods. Be extremely cautious and ask restaurants if they have a separate fryer for fries which is gluten-free.

fructose (fruit sugar) - 0

Fructose, or fruit sugar, is naturally gluten-free.

game - 0

Game meat, like venison or quail, is naturally gluten-free, provided it's not prepared with gluten-containing ingredients. (Dried game in the form of jerky or bars may well contain gluten)

garden cress - 0

Garden cress is naturally gluten-free.

garlic (usually well tolerated) - 0

Garlic is naturally gluten-free.

Geheimratskaese, Geheimrats cheese - 0

Geheimratskaese, or Geheimrat cheese, is typically gluten-free, but check labels to be sure.

German turnip - 0

German turnip, also known as kohlrabi, is naturally gluten-free.

ginger - 0

Ginger is naturally gluten-free.

glucose - 0

Glucose, a type of sugar, is naturally gluten-free.

goat's milk, goat milk - 0

Goat's milk is naturally gluten-free.

goji berry, Chinese wolfberry, Chinese boxthorn, Himalayan goji, Tibetan goji - 0

Goji berries are naturally gluten-free.

goose (organic, freshly cooked) - 0

Goose is naturally gluten-free, provided it is prepared and cooked without gluten-containing ingredients.

gooseberry, gooseberries - 0

Gooseberries are naturally gluten-free.

Gouda cheese (young) - 0

Young Gouda cheese is typically gluten-free, but check labels to be sure.

Gouda cheese, old - 0

Old Gouda cheese is typically gluten-free, but check labels to be sure.

gourds - 0

Gourds, like pumpkins and squash, are naturally gluten-free.

grapefruit - 0

Grapefruit is naturally gluten-free.

grapes - 0

Grapes are naturally gluten-free.

gravy - 1

Gravy, especially in restaurants and ready-made versions, often contains flour as a thickening agent, which contains gluten. However, it's possible to make gluten-free gravy using alternatives like cornstarch or gluten-free flour mixes. Always check labels if buying from the store, and inquire at restaurants. Homemade gravy can be easily controlled for gluten content.

green algae, algae - 0

Green algae is naturally gluten-free.

green beans - 0

Green beans are naturally gluten-free.

green peas - 0

Green peas are naturally gluten-free.

green split peas - 0

Green split peas are naturally gluten-free.

green tea - 0

Green tea is naturally gluten-free, but flavored or blended varieties may contain gluten, so check labels.

guava - 0

Guava is naturally gluten-free.

ham (dried, cured) - 1

Dried, cured ham can sometimes contain gluten due to flavorings or additives, so always check the label.

hazelnut - 0

Hazelnuts are naturally gluten-free.

hemp seeds (Cannabis sativa) - 0

Hemp seeds are naturally gluten-free.

herbal teas with medicinal herbs - 1

Herbal teas can sometimes contain gluten due to cross-contamination during processing or from added flavors. Check labels and consider the ingredients in the blend.

honey - 0

Honey is naturally gluten-free.

horseradish - 0

Horseradish is naturally gluten-free.

hot chocolate - 1

Hot chocolate can contain gluten, especially if it's pre-packaged or from a mix. Always check labels.

Indian fig opuntia, Barbary fig, cactus pear, spineless cactus, prickly pear, tuna - 0

These types of cactus fruits are all naturally gluten-free.

innards - 1

Innards, or offal, from animals are naturally gluten-free, but be aware of how they are prepared and cooked. Often they could be prepared with some sort of grain, hence our caution here.

inverted sugar syrup - 0

Inverted sugar syrup is naturally gluten-free.

ispaghula, psyllium seed husks - 0

Ispaghula, also known as psyllium seed husks, is naturally gluten-free.

Jeera (Cumin) - 0

Jeera, also known as cumin, is a spice that is naturally gluten-free. For extra safety, buy spices that are sold as a single ingredient spice, rather than a mix.

Jostaberry - 0

Jostaberry is a type of berry that is gluten-free.

Juniper Berries - 0

Juniper berries are naturally gluten-free.

Kaki (Persimmon) - 0

Kaki, or Persimmon, is a fruit that is naturally gluten-free.

Kale - 0

Kale is a leafy green vegetable that is naturally gluten-free.

Kefir - 0

Kefir, a fermented milk product, is generally gluten-free, but check labels for potential added ingredients. Some store bought brands may use non-gluten-free oats or other products containing gluten to add flavor or texture.

Kelp (Large Seaweeds, Algae) - 0

Kelp, a type of large seaweed or algae, is naturally gluten-free.

Kelp, Seaweed, Algae - 0

These are different types of sea vegetables and are naturally gluten-free.

Khorasan Wheat - 2

Khorasan wheat, also known as Kamut, is a type of wheat, which contains gluten.

Kiwi Fruit - 0

Kiwi fruit is naturally gluten-free.

Kohlrabi - 0

Kohlrabi is a type of vegetable that is naturally gluten-free.

Kombu Seaweed - 0

Kombu is a type of seaweed that is naturally gluten-free.

Lactose (Milk Sugar) - 0

Lactose is a type of sugar found in milk and is naturally gluten-free.

Ladyfinger Banana - 0

Ladyfinger bananas, like all bananas, are naturally gluten-free.

Lamb (Organic, Freshly Cooked) - 0

Freshly cooked, organic lamb is naturally gluten-free, but be cautious of any seasonings or marinades used.

Lamb's Lettuce, Corn Salad - 0

Both lamb's lettuce and corn salad are naturally gluten-free.

Langouste - 0

Langouste, also known as spiny lobster, is naturally gluten-free.

Lard - 0

Lard, a type of fat, is naturally gluten-free.

Laurel, Bay Laurel, Sweet Bay, Bay Tree, True Laurel, Grecian Laurel - 0

These are all names for the same plant, whose leaves are used as a seasoning and are naturally gluten-free.

Leek - 0

Leeks are a type of vegetable and are naturally gluten-free.

Lemon - 0

Lemons, like all fruits, are naturally gluten-free.

Lemon Peel, Lemon Zest - 0

Lemon peel and zest, like the fruit, are naturally gluten-free.

Lemonade - 1

While lemons are gluten-free, some commercially-prepared lemonades may contain gluten, so check labels carefully.

Lentils - 0

Lentils are a type of legume and are naturally gluten-free. However, they may be cross-contaminated during processing, so ensure they are labeled gluten-free.

Lettuce Iceberg - 0

Iceberg lettuce, like all types of lettuce, is naturally gluten-free.

Lettuce: Head and Leaf Lettuces - 0

All types of head and leaf lettuces are naturally gluten-free.

Lime - 0

Limes, like all fruits, are naturally gluten-free.

Lime Blossom Tea, Limeflower, Flowers of Large-Leaved Limetree - 0

Lime blossom tea and lime flowers are naturally gluten-free.

Lingonberry - 0

Lingonberries are a type of fruit and are naturally gluten-free.

Liquor, Clear - 1

Clear liquors can vary greatly in their gluten content depending on their ingredients and distillation process. Some are made from grains that contain gluten, so check labels carefully.

Liquor, Schnapps, Spirits, Cloudy (Not Colourless) - 1

Cloudy spirits and schnapps can contain gluten, especially if made from grains, so read labels carefully.

Liquorice Root - 0

Liquorice root itself is gluten-free, but processed liquorice sweets often contain gluten, so be sure to check labels.

Lobster - 0

Lobster, like all shellfish, is naturally gluten-free, but be aware of any potential sauces or seasonings.

Loganberry - 0

Loganberries are a type of fruit and are naturally gluten-free.

Lychee - 0

Lychee is a fruit that is naturally gluten-free.

Macadamia - 0

Macadamia nuts are naturally gluten-free.

Malt Extract - 2

Malt extract is made from barley, which contains gluten.

Malt, Barley Malt - 2

Malt, including barley malt, is made from barley, which contains gluten.

Maltodextrin - 1

Maltodextrin is a processed food ingredient. In the U.S., it is typically made from corn or potatoes and is gluten-free, but in Europe, it can be made from wheat, so check labels carefully.

Maltose, Malt Sugar (Pure) - 2

Maltose, also known as malt sugar, is made from barley, which contains gluten.

Mandarin Orange - 0

Mandarin oranges, like all fruits, are naturally gluten-free.

Mango - 0

Mangoes, like all fruits, are naturally gluten-free.

Maple Syrup - 0

Pure maple syrup is naturally gluten-free, but some brands may contain additives, so check labels.

Margarine - 1

While margarine is typically gluten-free, some brands may include additives or thickeners that contain gluten, so check labels carefully.

Marrow - 0

Marrow, a type of squash, is naturally gluten-free.

Mascarpone Cheese - 0

Mascarpone cheese is typically gluten-free, but check labels to ensure no gluten-containing additives have been used.

Mate Tea - 0

Mate tea is made from the naturally gluten-free yerba mate plant.

Meat Extract - 1

Meat extract can sometimes contain gluten due to added ingredients or flavorings, so always check the label. This is definitely one to be very cautious of

Melons (Except Watermelon) - 0

All melons, except watermelon, are naturally gluten-free.

Meridian Fennel - 0

Meridian fennel is a type of fennel and is naturally gluten-free.

Milk, Lactose-free - 0

Lactose-free milk is gluten-free, as milk itself does not contain gluten.

Milk, Pasteurised - 0

Pasteurised milk, like all milk, is naturally gluten-free.

Milk, UHT - 0

UHT, or Ultra High Temperature, milk is gluten-free.

Milk powder - 0

Milk powder is made from milk, which is naturally gluten-free.

Millet - 0

Millet is a type of grain that is naturally gluten-free.

Minced Meat (If Eaten Immediately After Its Production) - 0

Freshly minced meat is gluten-free, but be aware of any potential seasonings or additives.

Minced Meat (Open Sale or Pre-Packed) - 1

Pre-packaged minced meat can sometimes contain gluten due to added fillers or flavorings, so always check labels.

Mineral water, still - 0

Still mineral water is naturally gluten-free.

Mint - 0

Mint in its natural form is gluten-free.

Mold cheeses, mould cheeses - 1

Some mold cheeses are made with cultures that could contain gluten, so always check labels. The website *Beyond Celiac* tells us *'Some suggest that mold cultures of cheese may be grown on wheat or rye bread, so read the ingredients label. Generally, unless the ingredients label includes wheat, barley, rye or their derivatives, cheese should be safe.'*

Morel - 0

Morel mushrooms are naturally gluten-free.

Morello cherries - 0

Morello cherries are gluten-free in their natural state.

Mozzarella cheese - 0

Most mozzarella cheese is gluten-free but double-check for any additives on the label.

Mulberry - 0

Mulberries are naturally gluten-free.

Mungbeans (germinated, sprouting) - 0

Mungbeans are gluten-free, even when germinated or sprouted.

Mushrooms, different types - 0

Mushrooms of all types are naturally gluten-free.

Mustard, mustard seeds, mustardseed powder - 0

Mustard, its seeds, and powder are gluten-free, but check packaged mustards for additives.

Napa cabbage - 0

Napa cabbage is naturally gluten-free.

Nashi pear - 0

Nashi pears, like all pears, are naturally gluten-free.

Nectarine - 0

Nectarines are naturally gluten-free.

Nigella sativa oil - 0

Oil derived from Nigella sativa (black cumin) does not contain gluten.

Nigella sativa seed - 0

The seeds of Nigella sativa are naturally gluten-free.

Nori seaweed - 0

Nori seaweed is naturally gluten-free.

Nut grass - 0

Nut grass is a plant and does not contain gluten.

Nutmeg - 0

Nutmeg in its pure form is gluten-free.

Nutmeg flower - 0

The flower of the nutmeg plant does not contain gluten.

Nutmeg flower oil - 0

Oil derived from the flower of the nutmeg plant does not contain gluten.

Nuts - 0

Nuts in their natural, raw form are gluten-free. This includes pine nuts, pistachios, cashews, Brazil nuts, almonds, pecans, macadamia nuts, peanuts, walnuts, and other natural nuts. Be cautious with flavored nuts, which may contain gluten-containing additives. The same goes for pre-packaged nuts.

Oat drink, oat milk - 1

Oats themselves don't contain gluten, but are often contaminated with it. Check labels to ensure your oat milk is certified gluten-free.

Oats - 1

Oats don't contain gluten naturally but are often processed in facilities that also handle gluten-containing grains, leading to cross-contamination. In addition, many people with gluten sensitivity don't eat oats. This from the NHS website. *"Oats do not contain gluten, but many people with coeliac disease avoid eating them because they can become contaminated with other cereals that contain gluten."* Look for oats and oat products specifically labeled as gluten-free.

Olive oil - 0

Pure olive oil is naturally gluten-free.

Olives - 0

Olives are naturally gluten-free, but always check labels for any potential additives.

Onion - 0

Onions are naturally gluten-free.

Orange - 0

Oranges are naturally gluten-free.

Orange juice - 0

Pure orange juice is gluten-free, but always check labels for additives.

Orange peel, orange zest - 0

Orange peel and zest are gluten-free.

Oregano - 0

Oregano in its natural form is gluten-free.

Ostrich - 0

Ostrich meat is naturally gluten-free.

Ostrich (organic, freshly cooked) - 0

Freshly cooked organic ostrich is naturally gluten-free.

Oyster - 0

Oysters are naturally gluten-free.

Pak choi - 0

Pak choi, or bok choy, is naturally gluten-free.

Palm kernel oil - 0

Palm kernel oil is naturally gluten-free.

Palm oil, dendê oil - 0

Palm oil and dendê oil are naturally gluten-free.

Palm sugar - 0

Palm sugar is a natural sugar that does not contain gluten.

Papaya, pawpaw - 0

Both papaya and pawpaw are naturally gluten-free.

Paprika, hot - 0

Hot paprika is naturally gluten-free. Watch out for additives in seasonings.

Paprika, sweet - 0

Sweet paprika is naturally gluten-free. Watch out for additives in seasonings.

Parsley - 0

Parsley is naturally gluten-free.

Parsnip - 0

Parsnips are naturally gluten-free.

Passionfruit - 0

Passionfruit is naturally gluten-free.

Pasta (search individual ingredients, eg wheat, corn) - 2

Traditional pasta is made from wheat and contains gluten. There are gluten-free pasta options available made from other grains like corn and rice and pea, but always check labels to confirm they're gluten-free. In restaurants ask for gluten-free pasta to be cooked in separate water in a separate pot (important - this does not always happen.)

Paw paw - 0

Paw paw, another name for papaya, is naturally gluten-free.

Peach - 0

Peaches are naturally gluten-free.

Peanuts - 0

Peanuts are naturally gluten-free, but be cautious with pre-packaged or flavored peanuts, which may contain gluten-containing additives.

Pear - 0

Pears are naturally gluten-free.

Pear, peeled canned in sugar syrup - 1

Canned fruits can sometimes contain additives or be processed in facilities that handle gluten. Check labels to ensure they're gluten-free.

Pearl sago - 0

Pearl sago, a type of starch from certain palm stems, is gluten-free.

Peas (green) - 0

Green peas are naturally gluten-free.

Pea shoots - 0

Pea shoots, the young leaves of the pea plant, are naturally gluten-free.

Pepper, black - 0

Black pepper in its pure form is gluten-free.

Pepper, white - 0

White pepper is gluten-free.

Peppermint tea - 0

Peppermint tea is typically gluten-free, but always check labels to ensure there are no additives or flavorings that contain gluten.

Perennial wall-rocket - 0

Perennial wall-rocket, a type of herb, does not contain gluten.

Persian cumin - 0

Persian cumin, like all cumin, is gluten-free.

Persimmon - 0

Persimmons are naturally gluten-free.

Pickled cabbage - 1

While cabbage is naturally gluten-free, pickling processes and additives can introduce gluten. Always check labels.

Pickled cucumber - 1

Similar to cabbage, cucumbers are naturally gluten-free, but the pickling process can introduce gluten. Check labels.

Pickled gherkin - 1

Gherkins are gluten-free, but the pickling process may introduce gluten. Check labels.

Pickled vegetables - 1

While vegetables are naturally gluten-free, the pickling process and potential additives can introduce gluten. Check labels.

Pine nuts - 0

Pine nuts are naturally gluten-free.

Pineapple - 0

Pineapple is naturally gluten-free.

Pistachio - 0

Pistachios are naturally gluten-free.

Pitaya, pitahaya, dragon fruit - 0

All these names refer to the same fruit, which is naturally gluten-free.

Pizza base (search individual ingredients, eg wheat, corn) - 2

Traditional pizza bases are made from wheat and therefore contain gluten. However, gluten-free alternatives are available and are usually made from grains like corn and rice. Always check labels to ensure they're gluten-free.

Plaice - 0

Plaice, a type of flatfish, is naturally gluten-free.

Plantains - 0

Plantains are a type of fruit similar to bananas, and are naturally gluten-free.

Plum - 0

Plums are naturally gluten-free.

Pomegranate - 0

Pomegranates are naturally gluten-free.

Pomegranate juice - 0

Pure pomegranate juice should be gluten-free, but always check labels to ensure there are no additives or flavorings that contain gluten.

Popcorn (plain, popped) - 1

Plain popcorn that has been popped is gluten-free. Be careful with flavored popcorn, as it may contain gluten-containing additives.

Poppyseed - 0

Poppy seeds are naturally gluten-free.

Porcini mushrooms - 0

Porcini mushrooms are naturally gluten-free.

Pork - 1

Pork in its natural state is gluten-free. However, be wary of processed pork products, such as sausages or bacon, as they may contain gluten. Very many sausages contain gluten.

Pork (organic, freshly cooked) - 0

Freshly cooked organic pork is gluten-free.

Portabello mushrooms - 0

Portabello mushrooms are naturally gluten-free.

Potato - 0

Potatoes are naturally gluten-free.

Potato flour - 0

Potato flour, made from ground potatoes, is gluten-free.

Potato starch - 0

Potato starch is naturally gluten-free.

Prunes - 0

Prunes, which are dried plums, are naturally gluten-free.

Pumpkin - 0

Pumpkin is naturally gluten-free.

Pumpkin seeds - 0

Pumpkin seeds are naturally gluten-free.

Quail - 0

Quail meat is naturally gluten-free.

Quince - 0

Quinces are naturally gluten-free.

Quinoa - 0

Quinoa is a gluten-free grain. However, it's a good idea to buy quinoa that is labeled gluten-free to avoid cross-contamination.

Quinoa flakes - 0

Like quinoa itself, quinoa flakes are gluten-free. Always check for gluten-free labeling to avoid potential cross-contamination.

Rabbit - 0

Rabbit meat is naturally gluten-free.

Radicchio - 0

Radicchio, a type of leaf chicory, is naturally gluten-free.

Radish - 0

Radishes are naturally gluten-free.

Raisins - 0

Raisins, which are dried grapes, are naturally gluten-free.

Rapeseed oil - 0

Rapeseed oil is naturally gluten-free.

Raspberries - 0

Raspberries are naturally gluten-free.

Red cabbage - 0

Red cabbage is naturally gluten-free.

Red onions - 0

Red onions, like all onions, are naturally gluten-free.

Red pepper, bell pepper - 0

Red peppers or bell peppers are naturally gluten-free.

Redcurrants - 0

Redcurrants are naturally gluten-free.

Reindeer - 0

Reindeer meat is naturally gluten-free.

Rice - 0

All types of rice (white, brown, basmati, jasmine, etc.) are naturally gluten-free.

Rice bran oil - 0

Rice bran oil, which is extracted from the outer layer of rice, is gluten-free.

Rice cakes - 1

Rice cakes are typically gluten-free, but always check labels as they may contain additives or be processed in a facility that handles gluten.

Rice flour - 0

Rice flour is naturally gluten-free.

Rice milk - 0

Rice milk, made from milled rice and water, is typically gluten-free.

Rice noodles - 0

Rice noodles, made from rice flour and water, are typically gluten-free. Always check labels to ensure they're not processed in a facility that handles gluten, or a product that contains gluten.

Rice paper - 0

Rice paper, made from rice flour, salt, and water, is typically gluten-free.

Rice vinegar - 0

Rice vinegar, made from fermented rice, is typically gluten-free. Always check labels to ensure no gluten-containing additives are present.

Rosemary - 0

Rosemary is naturally gluten-free.

Runner beans - 0

Runner beans are naturally gluten-free.

Rutabaga, swede - 0

Rutabagas, also known as swedes, are naturally gluten-free.

Rye - 2

Rye is a grain that contains gluten and should be avoided on a gluten-free diet.

Safflower oil - 0

Safflower oil is naturally gluten-free.

Saffron - 0

Saffron is naturally gluten-free.

Sage - 0

Sage is naturally gluten-free.

Salmon - 0

Salmon is naturally gluten-free.

Sardines - 0

Sardines are naturally gluten-free. However, if they are canned or prepared with sauces or marinades, these could contain gluten, so always check labels.

Sauerkraut - 1

Sauerkraut is typically gluten-free as it's made from fermented cabbage, but always check labels to ensure there are no gluten-containing additives.

Scallop - 0

Scallops are naturally gluten-free.

Sea bass - 0

Sea bass is naturally gluten-free.

Sea bream - 0

Sea bream is naturally gluten-free.

Seafood (fresh, unprocessed) - 0

Fresh, unprocessed seafood is naturally gluten-free. Be cautious with processed or packaged seafood, as it could contain gluten-containing additives.

Seaweed - 0

Seaweed is naturally gluten-free.

Sesame oil - 0

Sesame oil is naturally gluten-free.

Sesame seeds - 0

Sesame seeds are naturally gluten-free.

Shallots - 0

Shallots are naturally gluten-free.

Sheep - 0

Sheep meat, also known as lamb or mutton, is naturally gluten-free.

Shiitake mushrooms - 0

Shiitake mushrooms are naturally gluten-free.

Shrimp - 0

Shrimp is naturally gluten-free.

Skimmed milk - 0

Skimmed milk is naturally gluten-free.

Sloe berries - 0

Sloe berries are naturally gluten-free.

Smoked fish (plain, no additives) - 0

Plain smoked fish with no additives is gluten-free.

Smoked meat (plain, no additives) - 0

Plain smoked meat with no additives is gluten-free. Be cautious with flavored or pre-packaged smoked meats, which may contain gluten-containing additives.

Soba noodles - 2

Soba noodles are traditionally made from buckwheat, which is gluten-free, but they often also contain wheat flour. Therefore, they're not safe for those on a gluten-free diet unless specifically labeled as gluten-free.

Sorbet - 1

Sorbet is typically gluten-free as it's usually made from fruit and sugar. However, some brands may use additives or thickeners that contain gluten, or may manufacture their products in a facility that also processes gluten-containing items, so it's important to check the labels.

Sorghum - 0

Sorghum is a grain that is naturally gluten-free.

Sorghum flour - 0

Sorghum flour, which is milled from sorghum grain, is naturally gluten-free.

Soy sauce - 2

Traditional soy sauce is made using wheat and is therefore not gluten-free. However, there are gluten-free versions available, often labeled as tamari sauce or gluten-free soy sauce.

Spaghetti squash - 0

Spaghetti squash is a type of winter squash that is naturally gluten-free.

Spinach - 0

Spinach is naturally gluten-free.

Split peas - 0

Split peas are naturally gluten-free.

Squash (all varieties) - 0

All varieties of squash are naturally gluten-free.

Star anise - 0

Star anise is a spice that is naturally gluten-free.

Stevia - 0

Stevia is a natural sweetener that is gluten-free.

Strawberries - 0

Strawberries are naturally gluten-free.

Sugar (white, brown, confectioner's) - 0

Pure sugar, whether white, brown, or confectioner's, is gluten-free. However, be aware that certain brands may process their sugar in facilities that also process gluten-containing products, so always check the label.

Sunflower oil - 0

Sunflower oil is naturally gluten-free.

Sunflower seeds - 0

Sunflower seeds are naturally gluten-free.

Sweet potatoes - 0

Sweet potatoes are naturally gluten-free.

Swiss chard - 0

Swiss chard is a leafy green vegetable that is naturally gluten-free.

Tangerines - 0

Tangerines are naturally gluten-free.

Tapioca - 0

Tapioca, which is derived from the root of the cassava plant, is naturally gluten-free.

Tapioca flour - 0

Tapioca flour, also known as tapioca starch, is naturally gluten-free.

Tarragon - 0

Tarragon is a herb that is naturally gluten-free.

Tea - 0

Pure, unflavored tea is gluten-free. However, flavored teas or teas with additives may contain gluten, so always check the label.

Thyme - 0

Thyme is a herb that is naturally gluten-free.

Tofu - 0

Plain, unflavored tofu is usually gluten-free as it's made from soybeans. However, flavored or processed tofu may contain gluten, so always check the label.

Tomatillos - 0

Tomatillos, a staple in Mexican cuisine, are naturally gluten-free.

Tomatoes - 0

Tomatoes are naturally gluten-free.

Trout - 0

Trout is naturally gluten-free.

Tuna (fresh) - 0

Fresh tuna is naturally gluten-free. However, canned or packaged tuna may contain gluten in the form of broth or other additives, so always check the label.

Turkey (fresh, unprocessed) - 0

Fresh, unprocessed turkey is naturally gluten-free. However, processed turkey products like sausages, patties, or deli meats may contain gluten, so always check the label.

Turmeric - 0

Turmeric is a spice that is naturally gluten-free.

Turnips - 0

Turnips are naturally gluten-free.

Vanilla extract - 1

Pure vanilla extract is typically gluten-free. However, some lower quality or imitation vanilla extracts may use grain alcohol, so always check the label.

Venison - 0

Venison, which is deer meat, is naturally gluten-free.

Vinegar (distilled white, balsamic, wine, apple cider) - 0

Distilled white vinegar, balsamic vinegar, wine vinegar, and apple cider vinegar are all naturally gluten-free. However, malt vinegar is not gluten-free as it's made from barley, a gluten-containing grain.

Walnuts - 0

Walnuts are naturally gluten-free.

Watercress - 0

Watercress is a leafy green vegetable that is naturally gluten-free.

Wheat - 2

Wheat is a grain that contains gluten and should be avoided on a gluten-free diet.

Wheatgrass - 2

While the actual grass of wheatgrass does not contain gluten, it can be easily cross-contaminated with the wheat grain, which does contain gluten. It's recommended that those with celiac disease or gluten intolerance avoid wheatgrass unless it's specifically labeled as gluten-free.

Whitefish - 0

Whitefish is naturally gluten-free.

Wild rice - 0

Despite its name, wild rice is not actually rice but a type of grass. It is naturally gluten-free.

Wine - 0

Most wines are naturally gluten-free as they're made from grapes. However, be aware that some dessert wines may contain gluten due to added flavorings or other additives.

Xanthan gum - 0

Xanthan gum, a common food additive, is naturally gluten-free. However, it can sometimes be derived from wheat, barley, or rye. While the final product should not contain gluten, those with severe reactions to gluten should only use products specifically labeled as gluten-free.

Yams - 0

Yams are naturally gluten-free.

Yogurt (plain, unflavored) - 0

Plain, unflavored yogurt is typically gluten-free. However, flavored or sweetened yogurts may contain gluten, so always check the label.

Zucchini - 0

Zucchini, also known as courgette, is naturally gluten-free.

Please note that while these ratings indicate the gluten content of the food in its natural, unprocessed state, many factors can introduce gluten into these foods. These can include cross-contamination in the field or during processing, additives or ingredients used in preparation, or the use of shared cooking surfaces or utensils. Always double-check labels and, when in doubt, ask the manufacturer or your server for more information.

CASE STUDIES

The Gluten-Free Adventurer's Gravy Mishap

Introduction:

In our first case study, we follow the journey of Sarah, a dedicated individual who adheres strictly to a gluten-free diet due to a diagnosed gluten intolerance. Sarah has successfully navigated the intricacies of gluten-free living, diligently avoiding gluten-containing foods. However, a seemingly innocuous encounter with gluten-laden gravy challenged her commitment and offered valuable lessons for the future.

The Gravy Mishap:

During a family Christmas gathering, Sarah unknowingly consumed a generous serving of gravy that contained gluten. Her Mum happily told her she could eat everything on the table. Unaware of its gluten content, she enjoyed the meal without suspicion. Half way through her Mum said, "why have you got that gravy? There's a separate gravy for you?". (She hadn't said that originally, or at least Sarah hadn't heard). The next day, Sarah experienced adverse symptoms, including digestive discomfort, fatigue, and brain fog. Frustrated, she knew the reason; the gravy!

Lessons Learned:

Sarah's experience taught her several important lessons about maintaining a gluten-free lifestyle. Firstly, she realized the criticality of always double-checking ingredients, especially when consuming dishes prepared by others. Even her Mum. She resolved to be more confident in expressing her gluten-free requirements and assertively seek gluten-free alternatives when necessary.

Case Study: Frustrating Restaurant Miscommunication

Introduction:

In this case study, we follow the story of Mark, who's committed to maintaining a gluten-free diet due to his gluten intolerance.

The Restaurant Incident:

Mark visited a nice restaurant near his house. He's been there before and the servers are normally pretty reliable. He informed the server about his gluten intolerance and specifically requested a gluten-free meal. The server assured him that the chosen dish would be prepared without gluten and would meet his dietary requirements. Trusting the server's expertise, Mark refrained from reconfirming his order when it arrived. Upon receiving his meal, Mark began eating without any suspicion. However, halfway through, the server came over, apologised, and said he'd subsequently double checked with the chef, and his dish was not gluten-free but contained traces of gluten in its seasoning.

Lessons Learned:

This incident taught Mark several valuable lessons regarding ordering gluten-free meals at restaurants. Mainly, Mark realized the significance of double-checking. Though he trusted the server's assurance, he acknowledged that an additional verification step would have been a good idea. Most times when he reconfirms an order on its arrival, servers roll their eyes and think he's being over-cautious. This proves that he is not being over cautious. He learned the importance of being assertive and proactive in confirming the gluten-free status of his dish, whether by requesting to speak directly with the chef or asking for written confirmation of the ingredients used.

Conclusion:

This case study serves as a reminder for individuals following a gluten-free diet to be proactive, thorough, and resilient in their efforts to ensure a safe and satisfying dining experience.

Case Study: Exploring Gluten-Free Baking with Cassava Flour and Rice Flour

Introduction:

In this case study, we delve into the story of Emily, an avid baker who developed a love for the art of baking. But then, horror, she's diagnosed as celiac! How could this be? She even grew up in a pizza restaurant? She has to throw out her cookbooks and start again.

The Transition to Gluten-Free Baking:

As Emily embraced her gluten-free lifestyle, she initially felt disheartened by the thought of giving up her beloved baking. However, her determination led her to explore alternative flours, seeking ways to continue indulging her passion while adhering to her dietary needs.

Emily's research led her to discover the versatility of cassava flour and rice flour in gluten-free baking. Excited by the prospect, she started experimenting with various recipes and adaptations, substituting traditional wheat flour with these alternative flours.

The Joy of Cassava Flour and Rice Flour:

Through her baking adventures, Emily discovered the unique qualities and joys that cassava flour and rice flour brought to her gluten-free creations. Cassava flour, derived from the root vegetable cassava, provided a light and fluffy texture to her baked goods. It imparted a mild, nutty flavor that enhanced the overall taste of her creations.

Similarly, Emily found that rice flour, made from finely ground rice grains, offered excellent binding properties and contributed to a tender crumb in her gluten-free baked treats. She experimented with different varieties of rice flour, such as white rice flour and brown rice flour, each imparting its own distinctive characteristics.

As Emily continued to bake with these alternative flours, she discovered a newfound sense of creativity and satisfaction. She successfully crafted gluten-free bread, muffins, cookies, and cakes that rivaled their gluten-containing counterparts. The joy and accomplishment she experienced with each successful batch motivated her to further explore the vast possibilities of gluten-free baking.

Conclusion:

Emily's gluten-free journey not only allowed her to embrace her passion for baking but also led her to discover the delightful world of cassava flour and rice flour. Through experimentation and perseverance, she unlocked the potential of these alternative flours, and - okay - it's a different sort of baking, but still enjoyable and most importantly she feels good after eating the fruits of her labor.

Printed in Great Britain
by Amazon

35815450R00056